613.71
V946a

AUG '03

SEP '03

DEC '08

amazing
arms

NOV MAR '05

JAN '10

OCT -- 2001

amazing arms

Get Toned Triceps,
Beautiful Biceps, and
Sexy Shoulders
in Just Minutes a Day!

MICHELE VOURLIOTIS

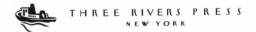

THREE RIVERS PRESS
NEW YORK

Published by Three Rivers Press, New York, New York.
Member of the Crown Publishing Group.

Random House, Inc. New York, Toronto, London, Sydney, Auckland
www.randomhouse.com

THREE RIVERS PRESS is a registered trademark and the Three Rivers
Press colophon is a trademark of Random House, Inc.

Printed in the United States of America

Design by Rhea Braunstein

*Illustrations on page 16 copyright © 2001 by
Nucleus Communications, Inc. All rights reserved.*

All other illustrations by Monica Rangne

Library of Congress Cataloging-in-Publication Data
Vourliotis, Michele.
Amazing arms : get toned triceps, beautiful biceps, and sexy shoulders
in just minutes a day! / Michele Vourliotis.—1st ed.
p. cm.
1. Arm exercises.   2. Shoulder exercises.
3. Exercise for women. I. Title.

GV508.V68 2001
613.7'1—dc21   2001023060

ISBN 0-609-80778-1

10   9   8   7   6   5   4   3   2   1

First Edition

CONTENTS

INTRODUCTION

As a personal trainer, I get many more questions like "How do I tighten up that jiggly part under my arm?" than "How can I improve my strength and stamina?" And even though the second question is more important than the first, the first is the truly burning question. The average person knows so much more about health and fitness than she did twenty-five years ago, the standards have changed.

Even though I still see plenty of people in the gym taking their first fitness steps, I see plenty more who are totally into the care and maintenance of their bodies. These people are not happy just to be fit—they want to see the cuts and curves and contours, the fruits of their labor. They see a picture of, say, Madonna's arms and think, "Yeah! That's what I want!" And I don't blame them—who doesn't want Madonna's arms?

Well, we may not share Madonna's genetics or the hours of personal training she can afford to devote to her body, but we can apply some of the same smart training techniques that got her to her ultra-buff status. It's not expensive, it's not complicated, it's not time-consuming. You do have to think lean and commit to a consistent program that zeroes in on the zone you want to hone. And you have to be prepared to stick with the program for at least six weeks to really see the magic. *Amazing Arms* will get you there—so let's get going!

amazing
arms

GETTING READY TO USE THIS BOOK

THERE'S almost nothing that suggests fitness the way toned, muscular arms do. When your arms and shoulders are in top form, you look capable and confident. And when they're not, we try to cover up, to camouflage and wish away our less than optimal arms. What a waste.

Why? Because your arms and shoulders are one of the easiest parts of your body to begin improving. Within weeks of focused attention on your arms, you can start to see real progress—a firming of the dreaded looseness and a definition around the curves and cuts of muscle. You'll even find yourself standing up straighter, as your posture and attitude respond to your physical development.

Put on a tank top and stand in front of the mirror,

hands on your hips. Are you wondering where those tight, toned arms you *used* to see in the mirror have gone? It's not as if you've been sitting around on the couch eating chips all this time. You carry groceries or a briefcase, you play golf or tennis, you vacuum—heck, you probably could have gold-medaled in the lifting-and-toting-toddlers competition at the Olympics. So why do you see slack instead of sleek? The answer is *time*.

Time changes your body and the lack of time challenges you to keep up with the changes your body is experiencing. You were probably at your muscular peak as a teenager, with a high ratio of muscle to fat, and a natural leanness and definition to your muscles. Every year that passes sees a decrease in muscle mass and strength, as well as an increase in body fat. The gradual loss of muscle mass is like gravity—it's happening naturally and without your permission. But it's compounded by diet, pregnancy, hormones, stress, and the level of physical activity you engage in—or not—regularly.

The good news is there are lots of smart, proactive things you can do to counter the effects of time, whatever your age, starting right now. And exercise is the number one smart, proactive thing you can do to bring your muscles back to where they once were—or where you've always wanted them to be. So what are you waiting for?

Now is the time to use this book to focus on bringing some strength and definition to your arms and shoulders. You're going to commit to following this book's recipes for amazing arms for a minimum of six weeks; and you're going to pay attention to the other important factors that affect your overall health and well-being, including aerobic exercise and diet.

Start Me Up

Here comes that old saw, the advisory warning you to consult your physician before beginning any fitness program. And we're not kidding. If you haven't done a lick of exercise since who knows when, you're overdue for an overview with your doctor. Use the exam and conversation as a motivational starting point for achieving the fitness goals you've outlined for yourself.

And if you have a healthy history, including a recent physical exam, moderate exercise, and a decent diet, and you just want to fine-tune, starting with your arms, let's do it! No matter which state you're starting from, though, start slowly so you can get to know your body's needs and limits and make the most of your *Amazing Arms* program.

BODY BASICS

BEFORE we attack the *Amazing Arms* program, it's good to get to know your arms first. In this book, we will be discussing exercises for the *triceps, biceps, shoulders,* and *forearms.* When you're aware of what your muscles look like, where they are, and how they work, it's a lot easier for you to visualize and execute the exercises to their best effect.

Triceps

The triceps is a three-headed muscle (hence its name, *triceps*) that is located at the back of your upper arm. Your triceps work to straighten your elbow and also to help your chest muscles when you push something. Often referred to as your *tris,* triceps do not get much

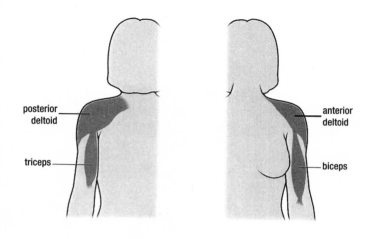

posterior deltoid

triceps

anterior deltoid

biceps

of a natural workout in daily life, which makes exercise especially important. Weak triceps are the cause of those jiggly arms that make you start thinking about wearing long-sleeved tops year-round.

Biceps

The biceps is a two-headed muscle (hence its name, *biceps*) that runs along the inside and front of your upper arm. The biceps are responsible for bending your arm at the elbow. Sometimes called *bis,* strong biceps are the signature element of a buff look. Gotta have 'em.

Shoulders

The deltoids (or *delts*) wrap completely around the tops of your arms and allow you to raise your arms forward, backward, and to the side, and to rotate inward and outward. This muscle group is divided into three parts: anterior delt (front), medial delt (side), and rear or posterior delt (back). Well-developed deltoids help you to avoid injuries such as shoulder dislocations or muscle tears.

Forearms

The forearm muscles consist of wrist extensors and flexors and run from the bottom of your elbow to your wrist. These muscles work to bend and move your wrists. Powerful forearms will give you a stronger grip for weight lifting, golf, or tennis, and will also help to prevent or alleviate ailments such as tennis elbow and carpal tunnel syndrome.

While these arm-related muscles and muscle groups are the focus of our attention here, keep in mind that they don't operate in a vacuum. Your back and chest, for example, have an intimate relationship with your shoulders. And your abdominals together with your back are the key to your posture and carriage. So I mean it when I say "abs tight" or "back strong" as we work through the *Amazing Arms* program—you won't get 100 percent out of it if you don't pay attention to these other factors.

TOOL BAG

You can get amazing arms with a minimum amount of time, space, and equipment. The only thing you really need to get started is a set of three-, five-, and eight-pound dumbbells. You might even consider including a two- and ten-pound weight in your set. Additional equipment and accessories, such as a workout bench or a body bar, aren't essential to these exercises but may help you get more out of your workout.

Dumbbells

A dumbbell, a short bar with weights attached to either end, can usually be held in one hand. For most of the exercises in this book, you will need two dumbbells, one for each hand. When purchasing dumbbells, you need to decide whether you want to purchase individual sets of dumbbells in two- or three-, five-, eight-, and ten-pound weights or an adjustable dumbbell kit. Either option has its advantages: Individual sets of dumbbells in the varied weight denominations that you need for the exercises in this book may be more convenient, but if you hope to eventually progress to lifting larger amounts of weight, an adjustable system allows for that.

Adjustable dumbbell kits usually sell for $30 to $100, depending on the brand, material they are made of, and quantity of attachable weights included in the kit. Individual sets of dumbbells in the three different weights usually sell for a total of between $20 and $100, again depending on the brand and material.

Plain metal dumbbells are the least expensive choice, costing from $20 to $40 for the three sets you need. Many people prefer rubber-coated dumbbells to plain metal dumbbells because they are easier to grip, invulnerable to rust, and perhaps more aesthetically pleasing. These are slightly more expensive, with a price range of $30 to $50 for the three sets. You can also buy chrome dumbbells, which are the most expensive, costing anywhere from $50 to $100 for the three sets, but they are also long lasting and very durable. Most professionals opt for chrome dumbbells.

H₂O

Because I'm on a big campaign to get people to drink more water and because you should never work out without it, you gotta have the water bottle. Get and use a bottle you'll fill and tote with you every time you work out.

Space

The exercises in this book do not require a lot of space. Many people like having a designated exercise space for workouts, in part because it helps them discipline themselves to work out regularly. But this isn't really necessary if you don't have the luxury of having your own little gym area. You can do these exercises almost anywhere in your home, or at the gym, of course. Just be sure you have enough clearance and that you're out of the path of traffic.

Extras

Although they are not necessary for achieving amazing arms, the following additional accessories might help motivate you and make your exercise routine as efficient and comfortable as possible.

Exercise Bench

A bench is a nice thing to have if you have the space and the inclination. It's built for just the kinds of dumbbell exercises we have in mind; it's sturdy, stable, and convenient. Flat basic benches cost from $45 to $100.

Exercise Mat

Exercise mats are made of foam, sometimes coated with some other material, such as latex or plastic. They are especially useful for any exercises or stretches that require that you use the floor. You might find that you want an exercise mat if you are uncomfortable being in direct contact with the floor. Exercise mats cost between $10 and $40.

Body Bar

This weighted bar can substitute for dumbbells at times, and some people swear by them for balance and even motion during strength training. They come in a variety of weights, from four to twenty-four pounds, and range in price from $20 to $50.

Gloves

Exercise gloves cover the palm of your hand and the lower parts of your fingers for a better grip on weights.

They are typically used only by serious weight lifters who are lifting large amounts, but if you have sensitive skin on your hands or tend to develop calluses, you may want to get a pair. The gloves usually sell for about $10 to $30.

Attire

Gym clothes are specially designed to provide extra flexibility and support during a workout. But you don't have to wear anything special to do these exercises, as long as your outfit is comfortable, allows full freedom of motion (especially for your arms and shoulders), and breathable. A sports bra is always a good idea. And do tie back your hair if it's long, as you don't want to be distracted (or entangled!) when you work out.

STRETCH THIS WAY

S TRETCHING is an important part of any workout. It improves flexibility, prevents soreness and stiffness after exercise, and lessens your risk of injury. Stretching takes only a few minutes and provides innumerable benefits to your body. No matter how little time you have, you should *never* skip stretching.

When to Stretch

The rule of thumb on stretching? *Never* stretch a cold muscle. So before you stretch—and then work out—you need to warm up for at least five minutes. Stretching after you have warmed up loosens your muscles and prepares you for your workout. Stretching after you exercise helps relax and elongate the muscles and may help prevent or reduce muscle soreness.

WARM UP!

Five minutes is all you need before stretching and working out. You can:

- walk, jog, or march in place
- walk or jog at 3.5 to 4 mph (or at a comfortable pace) on a treadmill
- pedal on a stationary (or regular!) bike

How to Stretch

Most experts agree that the best way to stretch is by easing into a stretch and holding it for ten to thirty seconds. You should feel a bit of tension, but not pain when you stretch. Short, rapid stretches can cause more harm than good, and often lead to injury, so this approach is not recommended. When stretching before a workout, the muscles you need to concentrate on are the ones you are going to use. It is fine to stretch other muscles as well, but remember to focus on the ones that will be working the most—in this case, your arms and shoulders.

Triceps

In a standing or sitting position, raise your right arm above your head. Bending the elbow, place your right hand behind your head. Your right hand should be resting just below your neck. Then, grip the elbow of your right arm with your left hand and pull toward the left gently, holding this stretch for ten to thirty seconds. Then repeat the stretch, this time putting your left hand behind your head, and using your right hand to pull your left.

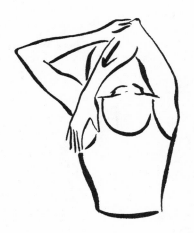

Biceps and Forearm

In a standing or sitting position, extend your right 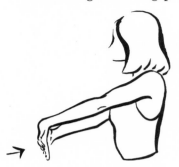 arm, palm facing up. With your left hand, gently press your palm back until you feel a stretch in your bicep and forearm. Hold for five seconds, then repeat with the other arm.

Shoulder and Chest

Hold on to both sides of a doorway with your hands behind you, as close to shoulder level as possible. Lean forward slightly, arms straight, chest up, and stretch gently for ten to thirty seconds. If you prefer, stretch one arm at a time in the same manner.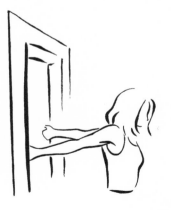

amazing arms

Deltoids

Using your left hand, gently pull your right elbow across your chest as far as is comfortable. Hold this stretch for ten to thirty seconds, then repeat the stretch with your left arm.

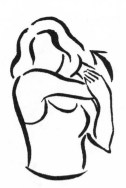

Deltoids and Chest

Keeping both arms straight, clasp them together behind your back. Pull them away from your back, as far as you possibly can without experiencing pain. Hold this stretch for ten to thirty seconds.

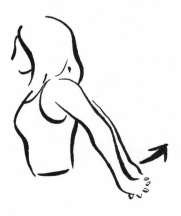

stretch this way

Shoulders

Relax your neck and slowly roll your shoulders up and backward in a circular motion five times. Repeat, moving your shoulders in the opposite direction (up and forward) five times.

A five-minute warm-up followed by these stretches will enhance your flexibility and enable a safe, effective workout. Don't even *think* about doing the *Amazing Arms* workout without it.

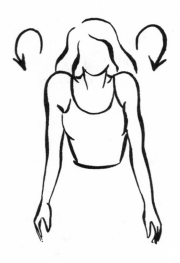

Upper Back

Interlace your fingers and hold your arms out in front of you, at shoulder height. Turn palms outward, extending arms forward, and hold for ten seconds.

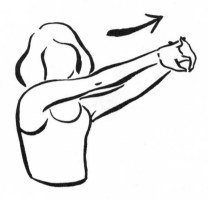

ARE WE THERE YET?

———

" THE Recipe for Amazing Arms," which follows this chapter, features the thirteen-plus exercises that will get you those amazing arms we've been talking so much about. But before we dig in, let's get a few important things straight.

Form Is Everything

As with all exercise, it's vitally important to pay close attention to your form when you perform these exercises. This ain't just for looks, folks. Proper form consists of good overall posture, correct positioning of the specific body parts in use, and correct positioning of the general body parts—usually head, shoulders, hips, and knees—that play a vital role in the execution of the exercise. Good form means getting 100 percent out of your effort. Good form also keeps your risk of injury at a minimum. In short, form counts.

Sign Up for the Program

Well, you bought this book, and that's very encouraging. But holding this book in your hands isn't what's going to get you those amazing arms. Committing to the *Amazing Arms* program for at least six weeks will. You need to find at least twenty minutes, three times a week, to do these exercises. And you need to find thirty more minutes or more, three or four days a week, to get your cardio in gear. Get out a calendar and mark off the days and time of day you are going to spend working on your arms. Try to plan to do your workout at the same time every time, so you're building an exercise habit while you're building strength and definition in your arms and shoulders. And plan to improve; besides the visible difference you'll see in your arms, you'll feel stronger and start thinking about increasing your weights or reps in order to challenge yourself more. But first, you have to commit.

Start at the Beginning

No matter what your physical condition, the first couple of times you do the *Amazing Arms* workout, you need to take it slow and easy, using a lesser weight and doing the minimum number of reps. Even though you're feeling enthusiastic as you start this new program, and may be tempted to go all out, it's important to pace yourself in the beginning because it allows you to learn the exercises and develop correct form. It also lets you determine any limitations you might have, or whether a certain combination of the exercises might work best for you. It's the getting-to-know-you (and your arms) stage of the *Amazing Arms* program.

When to Work Out

Put ten fitness professionals in a room and ask them what's the best time of day to work out and you'll get ten different answers. This is because there's no single right answer to this question. In part, it depends on *you*, your physical rhythms and realities. Are you a morning person or are you most engaged later in the day? Do you find it takes your body a while to get "warmed up" in the morning? Or to ask the most practical type of question, is 1:00 to 2:00 P.M. the only window of time you can steal while your toddler naps and your biggers aren't yet home from school? All of these considerations matter, and only you can decide what's the best time of day for you to spend on your soon-to-be amazing arms.

Some experts advocate morning workouts because it elevates your metabolism for an extended time, an obvious benefit. Others recommend late-afternoon/early-evening workouts because the body is warm and resilient, the muscles more flexible from a day of moving around. For me, it's morning—if I don't work out early it doesn't happen.

There's no right answer to the when-to-work-out question but I can tell you this with absolute certainty: Pick a time you can stick to. If early in the morning, before everyone in your household wakes up, is the time you can fully commit to, sign up for early-morning workouts. If you can't carve out time until after work, make 6:00 P.M. your target time. If you have to vary your workout time occasionally due to the shifting sands of daily life, by all means do so. But your best chance of sticking to your *Amazing Arms* program calls for a near religious commitment to the routine, which includes a regular time and place for working out.

Breathing, Reps, and Rest

Throughout the *Amazing Arms* exercises that follow, you need to remind yourself regularly to breathe. Seems like you shouldn't have to be reminded, but trust me, it's easy to accidentally hold your breath when exercising. The rule of thumb regarding breathing is exhale on the lift, inhale on the lower. But if you're making yourself crazy trying to inhale and exhale on the right beat, just breathe as you normally would. Whatever you do, though, don't hold your breath. Breathing ensures that oxygen is flowing to all points, especially your heart, as you exercise.

Just to clarify the shorthand, *reps* are the repetitions, or number of times you repeat the exercise. A *set* is number of reps you perform without stopping for a rest. So a set of ten reps is ten of the same exercise performed consecutively, to be followed by a brief period of rest before resuming a second set.

I'm firmly in the camp of trainers who believe that doing millions of sets of each exercise is *not* the way to get the most out of your workout. This approach is boring and time-consuming, creates the possibility of strain and injury, and is likely to cause your form to slip. Instead, focus on doing two clean, well-executed sets of each exercise, moving smoothly and efficiently from set to set. If you're focusing on your form, you're getting 100 percent out of your work. And if you're working efficiently, you're even getting some cardio action.

Rest between exercises and workouts is as important as the workouts themselves. You need to rest the recommended thirty seconds (or more if you're working with an increased weight) between sets so your muscles can recover enough for you to repeat the exercise or move on to the next. And you absolutely need to rest the muscle group you're working for a day or two between workouts. Don't try to cheat on rest, or you'll risk overexertion or, worse, injury.

Finally, you may feel a little sore after you begin the *Amazing Arms* regimen and this is to be expected. Do cardio work for a couple of days until the soreness disappears. Then resume the *Amazing Arms* program, working gently until your muscles become accustomed to the workout. If you've mistakenly pushed yourself to the point where you have a nagging discomfort that doesn't subside after a few days, stop the program and consult your doctor.

THE RECIPE FOR AMAZING ARMS
THIRTEEN EXERCISES TO TRIM AND TONE

WHAT follows are thirteen basic exercises that will make up your *Amazing Arms* program. Each exercise zeroes in on an important aspect of your arms and shoulders. Every workout will not consist of *all* of these exercises, but a combination of six or seven at a time that will hit on all the hot spots. The combos appear as menus directly following these exercises.

TRICEPS KICKBACK
(triceps)

Nice, tight, and focused, this neat little exercise is good for people at all levels and can be done on the floor or kneeling on a bench or a sturdy chair.

You'll Need
A bench or sturdy chair; 3-, 5-, 8-, or 10-pound dumbbell

Ready, Set
1. Kneel on a bench or sturdy chair with your left knee.
2. Place your left hand on the bench in front of you, back flat (picture yourself as a table), abs tight.
3. Keep your right foot on the floor with a slightly bent knee.
4. Hold the weight in your right hand, palm facing in.
5. Raise your elbow until your tricep is parallel with the floor.

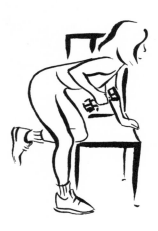

amazing arms

<u>*Go*</u>

6. Keeping your palm facing in and using your elbow as a hinge, slowly lift the weight behind you, keeping tricep stationary.
7. Slowly lower the dumbbell to your starting position.

<u>*Repeat*</u>

Complete a full set of 12 to 15 reps. Rest for at least 30 seconds, then switch sides and repeat.

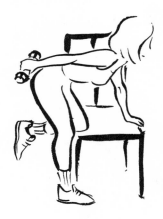

<u>*Don't Forget*</u>

■ Keep your triceps firm and close to your body. Breathe!
■ Do not swing your arm; use muscle, not momentum, to keep the weight moving.

the recipe for amazing arms

TRICEPS DIP
(triceps advanced)

A hit 'em where it works move, this classic exercise strengthens and sculpts the triceps. And since it requires no weight other than your own, it's a great exercise to do when you travel.

You'll Need
A bench or sturdy chair

Ready, Set
1. Sit on a bench or chair.
2. Place your palms on the bench on either side of your hips, knuckles facing forward.
3. Using your arms, lift your body off the bench and walk out until your legs form a 90-degree angle.

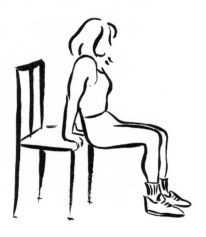

amazing arms

Go

4. Staying close to the bench or chair, bend your elbows and slowly lower your body toward the floor. Be careful not to hyperextend your shoulders.

5. Gently press your elbows up again, focusing on using your triceps.

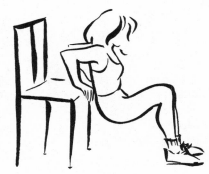

Repeat
Complete two full sets of 12 to 15 reps, resting for at least 30 seconds between sets.

Don't Forget
- No lockouts! Keep the elbows supple throughout the move. Breathe!
- Keep the focus on the triceps by maintaining 90-degree angles at the elbows and knees. If your posture sags, it's time to take a break.

BIGGIE THAT!
This exercise can be made more advanced by lifting one foot off the floor and balancing on one leg while doing the exercise. Or you can position your feet even farther away from your body to make the exercise more challenging.

the recipe for amazing arms   43

FACEBREAKER
(triceps)

This exercise is challenging, but if you keep with it, you'll learn a lot about control.

You'll Need
3-, 5-, or 8-pound dumbbells

Ready, Set
1. Lie on your back with your knees bent, feet flat on the floor.
2. Press your lower back into the floor while keeping your abdominals tight.
3. Holding a dumbbell in each hand, extend your arms straight up with palms facing your body.

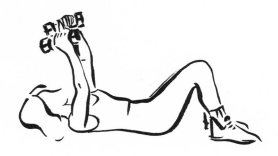

Go
4. Keeping your palms facing in and your elbows in place, slowly lower the dumbbells to the corresponding sides of your face.
5. Slowly lift the dumbbells until your arms are almost straight, back to the starting position.

　　　　amazing arms

Repeat

Complete two full sets of 12 to 15 reps, resting for 30 seconds between sets.

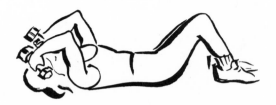

Don't Forget

- This exercise won't do you any good if you don't maintain total control over the movement. Don't let your arms swing or rely on momentum—make each repetition deliberate and controlled.
- Keep your triceps stationary and keep your elbows close in to take this movement through a full range of motion.

BICEPS CURL
(biceps)

The biceps curl tones and shapes the entire length of the biceps muscles—and gives you immediate gratification as you see and feel the muscles work.

You'll Need
3-, 5-, or 8-, or 10-pound dumbbells

Ready, Set
1. Stand with your feet hip-distance apart.
2. Slightly bend your knees, keeping your chest lifted and your abdominals tight.
3. With elbows glued to your sides, hold your weights in your hands, palms facing up.

Go
4. With your elbows close to your sides and your upper arms aligned with your body, curl dumbbells up toward your collarbone.
5. Maintaining the contraction, slowly lower the weights back down toward your starting position.

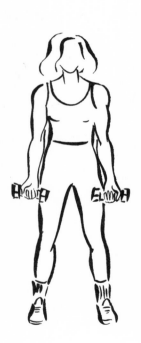

amazing arms

Repeat
Complete two full sets of 12 to 15 reps, resting 30 seconds between sets.

Don't Forget
- Keep your back straight; if you start to rock, you are using momentum, not muscle.
- Keep the focus on the biceps and don't lock the elbows.

WITH A TWIST!
You can do this exercise using one arm at a time, which lightens the load a bit for newcomers to arms workouts.

You can also do this exercise seated, being careful to maintain good posture.

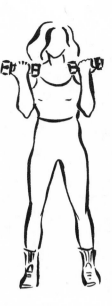

the recipe for amazing arms

21
(biceps)

21 is like your one perfect little black dress. It doesn't look like much on the hanger, but put it on, it makes an enormous impact. It's called 21 because you'll do seven reps at three different points of contraction. And it's all in the focus and technique.

You'll Need
3-, 5-, or 8-pound dumbbells

Ready, Set
1. Stand with your feet hip-distance apart.
2. Slightly bend your knees and keep your chest lifted.
3. Hold your weights at your sides, palms facing up. This is your first starting position.

Go
4. Keeping your elbows close to your sides and your upper arms aligned with your body, raise the weights so they are parallel with the floor.
5. Lower the weights to your starting position.
6. Repeat 7 times.
7. Next, raise the weights so they're parallel to the floor. This is your new starting position.
8. Slowly raise the weights toward your collarbone, keeping your elbows close to your sides.
9. Lower the weights to the parallel starting position.
10. Repeat 7 times.
11. Now lower the weights to the original starting position and do 7 deliberate bicep curls, lifting the weights for a full range of motion toward your collarbone.

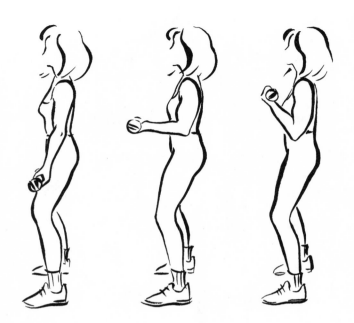

Repeat

Complete two full sets of 21 reps (7 reps from each of 3 positions), resting at least 30 seconds between sets.

Don't Forget

- Unlike the biceps curl, you must work both arms at the same time for this exercise.
- Make note of your start and stop points.
- Keep those elbows tucked into your sides.
- Stand up tall! Don't lean back or rock—use slow and controlled movements.

CONCENTRATED CURL
(biceps)

Also known as The Thinker, this exercise is a sophisticated little move that showcases your hard work.

You'll Need
3-, 5-, or 8-pound dumbbell; a bench or sturdy chair

Ready, Set
1. Sit on the end of the bench, your feet shoulder-width apart.
2. Holding a dumbbell in your left hand with your palm facing up, lean forward slightly and rest your left elbow against your left inner thigh.
3. Your free hand can rest comfortably on its corresponding leg.

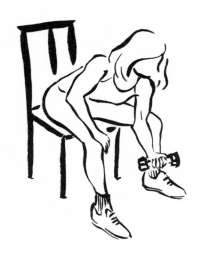

4. Keeping your elbow steady, slowly lower the weight toward the floor without losing the contraction.
5. Lift the weight toward your left shoulder, leaving your elbow resting against your leg.

Repeat

Complete a full set of 12 to 15 reps and switch arms. Do two sets for each side, resting for at least 30 seconds between sets.

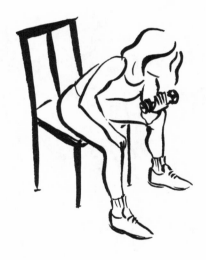

Don't Forget

■ Keeping your elbow pressed against your thigh will keep the movement steady and the biceps focused.

FRONT SHOULDER RAISE
(anterior deltoids)

This is officially called the anterior raise, but I like to call it the Tank Top Trimmer! This move works the front of your shoulders, priming them for—you guessed it—tank tops.

You'll Need
3-, 5-, or 8-pound dumbbells or an 8-, 10-, or 12-pound body bar

Ready, Set
1. Stand with your feet shoulder-width apart, knees soft, abs tight, chest lifted, shoulders down and back.

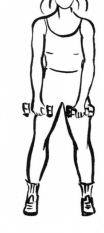
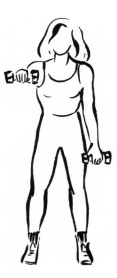

Go
2. Thinking of your arm as a lever and the shoulder as its hinge, raise the weight in your right hand to shoulder level, keeping your arm straight.
3. Slowly lower the weight to the starting position. Repeat with your left arm for one complete rep.

amazing arms

Repeat
Complete two full sets of 12 to 15 reps, resting at least 30 seconds between sets.

Don't Forget
- Use slow, controlled movements—no swinging, no momentum.
- Use less weight than you think you can handle the first time around, then increase the weight as you become accustomed to the exercise.

WITH A TWIST!
You can lift both arms together—rather than alternating—just be careful to make it a single, controlled movement.

This exercise can also be done sitting in a chair, lowering the weights to the sides of the chair.

LATERAL RAISE
(lateral deltoids)

This exercise works the sides of the shoulder and contributes to that nice cut you see on arms you admire.

You'll Need
3-, 5-, or 8-, or 10-pound dumbbells

Ready, Set
1. Stand with your feet shoulder-width apart, knees soft, abs tight, chest lifted, shoulders down and back.
2. Hold a dumbbell in each hand, palms facing in.

Go
3. With your elbows soft, lift the dumbbells to shoulder level and pause at the top.
4. Slowly lower the weights back down to the starting position.

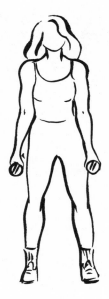

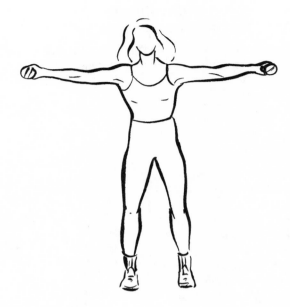

Repeat

Complete two full sets of 12 to 15 reps, resting at least 30 seconds between sets.

Don't Forget

■ Maintain good posture and careful control over the movement—no swinging, no momentum.

WITH A TWIST!

If you're a newcomer to arms action, try this exercise alternating arms at first, working up to doing both arms together. Or lift the weight with bent rather than straight arms when you first start out.

UPRIGHT ROW
(anterior, posterior, and lateral deltoids)

This exercise is good if you don't have a lot of time to work out because it hits all three parts of the shoulder.

You'll Need
3-, 5-, or 8-, or 10-pound dumbbells or 8-, 10-, or 12-pound body bar

Ready, Set
1. Stand with your feet hip-distance apart, knees slightly bent.
2. Keep your chest lifted and your abdominals in.
3. Hold the weights (either the dumbbells or the bar) at the front of your thighs, arms extended down, elbows soft, palms facing in.

Go
4. Keeping the weights close to your body and just a few inches apart (or holding the body bar with a narrow grip of just a few inches apart), pull the weights straight up toward your chest and hold for 2 seconds. Your body should form a T shape.

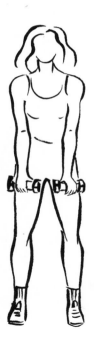

amazing arms

5. Slowly lower the weights to the starting position.

Repeat
Complete two full sets of 12 to 15 reps, resting at least 30 seconds between sets.

Don't Forget
■ Keep your wrists firm and positioned above the weights.

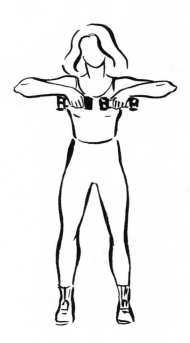

the recipe for amazing arms

THE PULSE
(posterior deltoids)

Say *sayonara* to slouching shoulders. This subtle move pulls the shoulder up and back, keeps the spine erect, and helps you remember what it feels like to stand tall.

You'll Need
3-, 5-, or 8-pound dumbbell

Ready, Set
1. Stand with your feet hip-distance apart, knees soft and slightly bent.
2. Keep abdominals tight, pelvis tucked, chest lifted, shoulders down.
3. With both hands, hold a single dumbbell behind you, placing the knobs of the dumbbell in each hand, palms facing out. The dumbbell should be horizontal to the floor.

Go
4. Working within a tiny range of motion, lift the weight no more than 6 or 8 inches away from your body and hold for a second.

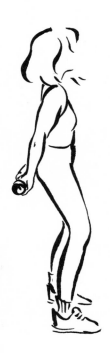

5. Lower the weight to the starting position.

Repeat
Complete two full sets of 12 to 15 reps, resting at least 30 seconds between sets.

Don't Forget
- Don't jerk or snap the weight—the movement should be smooth.
- Focus on bringing your shoulder blades together.

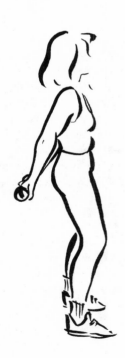

HAMMER CURL
(biceps and forearm)

As you do this one, pretend that you are actually holding a hammer.

You'll Need
3-, 5-, or 8-, or 10-pound dumbbells

Ready, Set
1. Stand with your feet shoulder-width apart, knees slightly bent.
2. Keep your abs tight, shoulders down, chest lifted.
3. Hold the dumbbells in your hands with palms facing in, hands down by your sides.

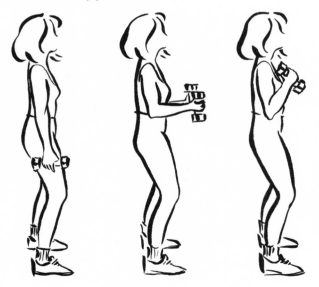

Go

4. Slowly raise the weights, hammer style, toward your shoulders, keeping your elbows stationary and close to your body.

5. Slowly lower the weights, careful not to lock your elbows.

Repeat

Complete two full sets of 12 to 15 reps, resting at least 30 seconds between sets.

Don't Forget

■ Keep your arms pressed close to your body.

WITH A TWIST!

You can alternate arms rather than lifting them together. Listen to your body and do what works best for you.

FOREARM CURLS

Fine-tuning your forearms is the icing on the cake of your arms workouts. This move works the front of your forearm, which is important for gripping.

You'll Need
2- or 3-pound dumbbell; a bench or sturdy chair

Ready, Set
1. Sit on the edge of a chair or a bench, keeping feet shoulder-width apart.
2. Lean your upper body slightly forward, keeping your chest lifted and back strong.
3. Hold the weight in your left hand with palm facing up.
4. Rest your left forearm on your left thigh with your wrist slightly beyond your knee.
5. Place your right hand comfortably on your right thigh.

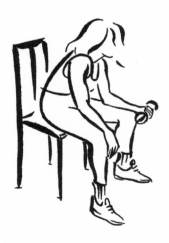

amazing arms

Go

6. Keeping your arm firm, curl the weight up toward your body and hold for 1 second.
7. Slowly lower the weight to the starting position.

Repeat

Complete a full set of 12 to 15 reps and switch arms. Do two sets for each side, resting for at least 30 seconds between sets.

Don't Forget

■ Keep the forearms firmly positioned on the thighs.
■ Isolate the movement so that your wrist is the hinge and no other part of your arm or body is moving.

REVERSE FOREARM CURLS

Works the back of your forearms. We leave no stone unturned.

You'll Need

2- or 3-pound dumbbell; a bench or sturdy chair

Ready, Set

1. Sit at the edge of a chair or a bench, feet shoulder-width apart.
2. Lean your upper body slightly forward, keeping your chest lifted.
3. Hold the dumbbell in your left hand with palm facing down.
4. Rest your left forearm on your left thigh with your wrist slightly beyond your knee.
5. Place your right arm comfortably on your right thigh.

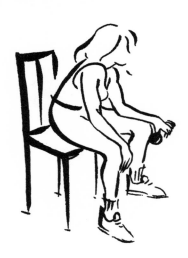

amazing arms

Go

6. Keeping your arm firm, curl the dumbbell down slowly toward the floor, holding for 1 second.
7. Slowly return the dumbbell to the starting position.

Repeat

Complete a full set of 12 to 15 reps and switch arms. Do two sets for each side, resting for at least 30 seconds between sets.

Don't Forget

- Keep the forearms planted on the thighs.
- For balance, always do forearm curls and reverse forearm curls together.

THE SQUEEZE

A great exercise for the forearms that no one needs to know you're doing.

You'll Need
A small rubber ball, a tennis ball, crumpled piece of paper, anything palm-sized and round.

Ready, Set
1. Standing or sitting, hold the item in your right hand.

Go

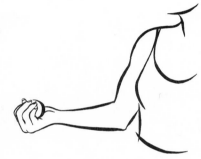

2. Squeeze and release, breathing steadily and evenly, as many times as you can.

Repeat
Switch hands and do it all over again.

Don't Forget
- Throughout exercise, be sure to maintain normal breathing—don't hold your breath.
- Keep a ball in your car and do this exercise while you wait at stoplights.

THE ABCS OF AMAZING ARMS

H ERE are the very basic guidelines for executing and mastering the exercises in the *Amazing Arms* program:

- Learn each exercise well, careful to perform it correctly every single time and with proper form.
- Don't use momentum; instead use a deliberate, consistent speed of movement. Cheating the exercise by using momentum takes the work away from your muscles and is, frankly, a waste of your valuable time.
- Use a full range of motion on every exercise.
- Keep your head completely focused on the muscle that you're working.

- Briefly stretch the major muscle groups between sets. This helps flexibility and muscle recovery.
- When you discover that the weight feels too light, it's time to move up to the next weight level. Or stick to the original weight level and execute the movement more slowly.
- Keep rest periods to no more than thirty seconds or so in order to keep your heart rate up and the effort efficient.

THE MENUS

FOLLOWING are the two combinations of *Amazing Arms* exercises to follow. You'll do Menu # 1 for weeks 1 through 3 and Menu #2 for weeks 4 through 6.

This approach will allow your body to "learn" each exercise to its maximum effectiveness, while providing a variety that challenges you differently over the course of the program. You will also learn the combinations well enough to incorporate into your future workouts, and can mix and match the exercises you like the best.

Menu #1

Triceps Kickback
Facebreaker
Biceps Curl
Concentrated Curl
Front Shoulder Raise
Lateral Raise
The Pulse
Forearm Curl
Reverse Forearm Curl
The Squeeze

Menu #2

Triceps Dip
Facebreaker
"21"
Hammer Curl
Upright Row
Front Shoulder Raise
Lateral Raise
Forearm Curl
Reverse Forearm Curl
The Squeeze

amazing arms

The Daily Drill

As with every training program focused on a single area of the body, you must adhere to the day-on/day-off rule so your muscles can heal between outings. Use the day off to focus on your aerobic effort. Because, as we'll discuss shortly, your arms are not alone in the quest for amazing arms.

YOUR ARMS ARE NOT ALONE

WHENEVER you undertake an exercise program, you bring your own history and genetics to the table—say, a predisposition to gain weight (store fat) in a certain area ("But I have my mother's hips!") or an energetic metabolism or even more serious matters, such as a family history of high blood pressure. These are your body basics—the facts about your anatomy, physiology, and history that can affect your success with any fitness program, including *Amazing Arms*.

In other words, it's not just your arms and the *Amazing Arms* exercises that'll get you where you want to go. You need to be prepared to ramp up your physical activity level, bringing in more everyday exertion and aerobic effort. And you need to pay attention to what's going on with your diet. This boils down to two rules that provide powerful backup to your *Amazing Arms* program: Be Active and Eat Right.

Be Active

When we talk about being active, we're talking about getting ourselves to the aerobic level in any number of physical activities. Aerobic means "with oxygen," so an aerobic (or cardiovascular) exercise is any activity that requires your body to use more oxygen—as well as an increase in resting heart rate and blood flow—during its performance. Regular aerobic activity is an essential element of any weight-training program, including (and especially!) *Amazing Arms.*

It's amazing how many routine tasks we perform every day without even thinking twice about the energy (and calories) we spend doing them. Washing a car, mowing the lawn, shoveling snow, and vacuuming—these familiar activities are great examples of ways you are active (and aerobic!) in your daily routine. So do these things whenever you have the chance—in fact, do more of them, or for longer, and soon you will have turned this higher level of day-to-day activity into a good, healthy habit.

The key to everyday exercise is to remember that it's always better to move than to be still. When watching television, don't lie down on the couch but sit up straight, getting up regularly to stretch or move around. Or better yet, don't sit on the couch at all; instead, get down on the floor and do some crunches as you watch TV. If you work in an office, don't sit at your desk for hours on end; instead, walk around and stretch well for a few minutes every hour or so. And try to spend half of your lunch hour walking—outside in the neighborhood, up and down the hallways, or even up and down stairs.

Remember that in order to lose a pound of fat, you must burn 3,500 calories. Naturally, the more active you are, the more calories you burn. Don't obsess over this fact. Just change your daily routine in little ways that add up, over time, to a lot. Park as far away from the entrance to the grocery store as you can and walk. Take your dog for a brisk twenty-minute outing instead of just a drag to the corner to do his business. Think of all the ways you can spend five minutes here and fifteen minutes there doing more of what you're doing already. And then do it.

Average Calories Burned During Household Activities

Household Activity	Average Calories Burned per 10 Minutes
Shoveling snow	125
Washing the walls	100
Painting the walls	90
Washing the car	90
Mowing the lawn	85
Washing the dog	65
Trimming the hedges	50
Weeding the garden	48
Cleaning the windows	40
Mopping the floor	38
Polishing the floor	38
Vacuuming	35
Raking	35
Dusting	30

Join Up!

Beyond the little ways you can ramp up your activity level on a day-to-day basis, you can always take this opportunity to join forces with other like-minded folks. Take a dance or yoga class once a week. Swim laps for an hour at the local pool every weekend. Get out there with your kids and ride bikes, Rollerblade, or hike. Do something way out of the ordinary for you—maybe join a kickboxing class or a runner's club. Joining a group always enhances your sense of commitment to the activity. Make a date with yourself by putting these activities on your calendar. Besides the dramatic physical benefits of taking up a new activity, the mental benefits of exploring a new activity and physical challenge are immeasurable. Do it—I dare you.

Average Calories Burned During Aerobic Activities

Aerobic Activity	Average Calories Burned per 20 Minutes
Running an 8-minute mile (outdoors or on a treadmill)	230
Running a 9-minute mile (outdoors or on a treadmill)	220
Cross-country skiing	220
Swimming	210
Kickboxing	200
Doing step aerobics	200
Stair-stepping	200
Rope jumping	200

(continues)

Aerobic Activity	Average Calories Burned per 20 Minutes
(continued)	
Doing low-impact aerobics (aerobic dance)	200
Nordic Track cross-country skiing	165
Trampoline jumping	165
Racewalking	160
Hiking (hills)	160
Rowing on a machine	150
Jogging at a slow pace (outdoors or on a treadmill)	145
Bicycle riding (stationary or moving at moderate pace)	140
Doing pool aerobics and water walking	140
Dancing at a quick pace	120
Walking at a quick pace (outdoors or on a treadmill)	110

The Art of Eating Right

You'd be surprised how many people believe that if you're exercising regularly, it doesn't matter what you eat. WRONG! If you exercise, it matters even more what you eat. When you engage in a regular exercise regime and don't pay attention to what you're eating, you're not going to get the results you're looking for. Further, if you exercise a nutrient-deficient body, you're not making it healthier; you're actually creating a more serious nutrient deficiency. To build a lean, strong body, what you eat *is* important.

We're not talking about "going on a diet" and restricting the amount and types of foods you eat, but rather tending to your diet and perhaps making adjustments that maximize your overall effort to improve your fitness. In short, the challenge is to balance the nutrient levels of the foods you eat.

Every body is different, and every body spends and stores in a different way. So the appropriate amount and combination of foods to eat is different for each of us. There are, however, some universal rules for eating healthfully.

• Cut back on salt. Too much salt can lead to water retention, which in the short term can lead to weight gain. And for those with a history of hypertension and/or who are salt sensitive, too much salt can contribute to or aggravate hypertension.

• Cut back on caffeine and alcohol. Both can lead to dehydration, which is the opposite of what your body needs and wants at all times. Further, they can act as stimulants that can confuse your goals and impulses, causing you to eat more food than you should or to eat foods that you should be avoiding.

• Drink a minimum of two liters of cold water a day, and more if possible. Your body will perform more effectively inside and out, it will help you manage your diet, and, as an added benefit, your skin will look better than ever. TIP: Drink 75 percent of your water intake goal before 5:00 P.M. if you can.

• Eat small meals, five times a day. This approach to eating spreads out your consumption more evenly over the course of the day, providing a steady stream of energy. Bigger meals are harder for your body to digest and can interrupt your energy level and mood rather than enhance it.

KEEP TRACK!

THIS is a template for the record you should keep of your *Amazing Arms* program, as well as the other activities you take up to enhance the effects of the program. Use this schedule to keep track of your progress, and as a place to note what you're doing dietwise to help yourself along. Note how much weight you're using and how many reps you're doing of each exercise. If it's an off day, write "off." Estimate how much time you spend on everyday activity as well as on focused aerobic exercise. Finally, try to summarize what you've eaten each day, to give you a picture of what you're really consuming and a place to start making adjustments.

Chart Your Progress

	MON	TUES	WED	THUR	FRI	SAT	SUN
Week #1							
Menu #1							
Triceps Kickback							
Facebreaker							
Biceps Curl							
Concentrated Curl							
Front Shoulder Raise							
Lateral Raise							
The Pulse							
Forearm Curl							
Reverse Forearm Curl							
The Squeeze							
Everyday Activity							
Aerobic Activity							
Diet Diary							

amazing arms

Chart Your Progress

	MON	TUES	WED	THUR	FRI	SAT	SUN
Week #2							
Menu #1							
Triceps Kickback							
Facebreaker							
Biceps Curl							
Concentrated Curl							
Front Shoulder Raise							
Lateral Raise							
The Pulse							
Forearm Curl							
Reverse Forearm Curl							
The Squeeze							
Everyday Activity							
Aerobic Activity							
Diet Diary							

Chart Your Progress

	MON	TUES	WED	THUR	FRI	SAT	SUN
Week #3							
Menu #1							
Triceps Kickback							
Facebreaker							
Biceps Curl							
Concentrated Curl							
Front Shoulder Raise							
Lateral Raise							
The Pulse							
Forearm Curl							
Reverse Forearm Curl							
The Squeeze							
Everyday Activity							
Aerobic Activity							
Diet Diary							

amazing arms

Chart Your Progress

	MON	TUES	WED	THUR	FRI	SAT	SUN
Week #4							
Menu #2							
Triceps Dip							
Facebreaker							
"21"							
Hammer Curl							
Upright Row							
Front Shoulder Raise							
Lateral Raise							
Forearm Curl							
Reverse Forearm Curl							
The Squeeze							
Everyday Activity							
Aerobic Activity							
Diet Diary							

Chart Your Progress

	MON	TUES	WED	THUR	FRI	SAT	SUN
Week #5							
Menu #2							
Triceps Dip							
Facebreaker							
"21"							
Hammer Curl							
Upright Row							
Front Shoulder Raise							
Lateral Raise							
Forearm Curl							
Reverse Forearm Curl							
The Squeeze							
Everyday Activity							
Aerobic Activity							
Diet Diary							

amazing arms

Chart Your Progress

	MON	TUES	WED	THUR	FRI	SAT	SUN
Week #6							
Menu #2							
Triceps Dip							
Facebreaker							
"21"							
Hammer Curl							
Upright Row							
Front Shoulder Raise							
Lateral Raise							
Forearm Curl							
Reverse Forearm Curl							
The Squeeze							
Everyday Activity							
Aerobic Activity							
Diet Diary							

INDEX

ABOUT THE AUTHOR

Michele Vourliotis is a certified personal trainer with specialties in weight training, spinning, and kick boxing. She is also the founder of the women's fitness program "Camp Mom." She lives with her family in Westchester County, New York.